All scripture references taken from the KJV of the Holy Bible unless otherwise indicated.

<u>Warfare Prayers Against Beauty Curses:</u>

<u>Sleep Pretty & Heal</u>, by Dr. Marlene Miles

Freshwater Press 2023

ISBN: 978-1-960150-60-8

Contents

Sleep Pretty 7

Beauty Rest...10

Men 14

Healing Sleep...15

Warfare..17

Fat Demons...22

Gut Health 24

Warfare 2...31

Pool of Siloam..35

Hear This 40

Diabetes 43

Asthma...50

Backache & Neckache 56

Healing Covenant..61

Inflammation & Infection 63

High Blood Pressure 64

Cancer..66

Headache 69

Reverse Beauty Curses & Skin Issues 71

Women's Disorders 80

Men's Disorders 85

Kidney & Liver 90

Healthy Sleep Positions 92

Facial Diseases..97

Emotions 106

Brain & Mind...109

Dear Reader 118

Other books by this author 118

Warfare Prayers Against
Beauty Curses
Sleep Well & Heal

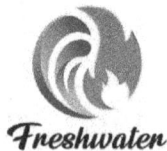

Freshwater

Freshwater Press, USA

I sleep pretty.

I rest well.

I get my beauty rest.

Lord, heal me in the night hours

while the night is quiet

and my body is still,

in the Name of Jesus.

Sleep Pretty

I sleep pretty. I rest well. I get my beauty rest. Lord, heal me in the night hours while the night is quiet, and my body is still, in the Name of Jesus.

Lord God, thank You that You love me. You invite me into Your presence where there is fullness of joy.

Free my body, soul, and spirit from any and all captivity of the devil and his entities, so that everything about my mind, soul, body, and spirit will be healed and made whole, in the Name of Jesus.

Touch me, Lord, inhabit my life and my being, and keep all evil away from me, in the Name of Jesus.

I bear in my body the marks of the Lord Jesus Christ. Satan, do not touch me, do not touch any part of me--, not my soul, not my spirit, not my body, in the Name of Jesus. Hands off!

O give thanks unto the Lord, call upon his name, make known his deeds among the people. Sing unto him. Sing songs unto him. Talk ye of his wondrous works. Glory in his holy name, let the heart of them rejoice that seek the Lord and his strength, seek His face continually.

Remember his marvelous works that he had done, his wonders, and the judgments of his mouth. He is the Lord our God, his judgments are in all the Earth.

Be mindful always of his covenant, the word which he commanded to thee a thousand generations. Even of the covenant which he made with Abraham and his oath unto Isaac, and have confirmed the same to Jacob, for a law and to Israel, and for an everlasting covenant. Sing unto the Lord all the earth show forth from day-to-day his salvation.

Declare his glory among the heathen his marvelous works among the nations. For great is the Lord, and greatly to be praised. He also is to be feared above all gods. For all the gods of the people are idols, but the Lord made the heavens.

Glory and honor are in his presence. Strength and gladness are in his place.

Give unto the Lord, ye kindreds of the people, give unto the Lord glory and strength give unto the Lord the glory due unto His name.

Bring an offering and come before him. Worship the Lord in the beauty of His Holiness. Fear before him all the earth. The world also shall be stable, that it be not moved.

Let the heavens be glad, and let the earth rejoice, and let men say among the nations the Lord reigns.

Let the sea roar, and the fullness thereof, let the fields rejoice in all that is therein. Then shall the trees of the woods sing out at the presence of the Lord, because he cometh to judge the earth.

Oh give thanks unto the Lord, for he is good, for his mercy endures forever.

And say, save us, O God, of our salvation, and gather us together and deliver us from the heathen. And we may give thanks to thy holy name and glory, and thy praise. Blessed be the Lord God of Israel, forever and ever. All the people said Amen. And praised the Lord. (1 Chronicles 16)

Beauty Rest

I sleep pretty. I rest well. I get my beauty rest.

Lord, heal me in the night hours when the night is quiet and while my body is still, in the Name of Jesus.

Lord God, thank You that You love me. You invite me into Your presence where there is fullness of joy.

Lord, give me healthy breathing, heal me from sleep apnea and snoring, so I rest well, and I sleep pretty.

Oh, show the people and the princes her beauty, for she was fair to look on. I am black, but comely o ye daughters of Jerusalem, as the tents of Kedar, As the curtains of Solomon. Thy cheeks are comely with rows of jewels, thy neck with chains of gold. (Song 1)

Lord, give me length of days. My life, body, and soul are preserved from premature deterioration. Thank You, Lord.

I age gracefully. My beauty shall not depart.

Deck thyself now with majesty and excellence, and array thyself with the glory and beauty.

Father, give me beauty for ashes, love for hate, gladness for mourning, peace for despair.

Make my heart glad, Lord, sing like the morning. Beautiful like the dawn. Fresh, like a new day. And the glorious beauty of the Lord.

Make me beautiful, Lord, in Your eyes. Thank You, Lord.

If the Lord does not glory in your beauty, it is in vain; it is vain glory.

If you do not glorify the Father in Your beauty, it is selfish and vain.

Lord, make me beautiful on the inside and the outside, in the Name of Jesus.

Appoint unto me beauty for ashes, the oil of joy for mourning, the garment of praise for the *spirit of heaviness*, Lord, that I might be called a tree of righteousness, the planting of the Lord, that You, Lord, will be glorified.

Restore me to health. Thank You, Father.

God gives rest to His beloved. I am beloved of God.

And He has put all my sins behind His back.

Thank You, Lord, for renewing my strength. Lord, You are the strength of my life. How great is Your goodness, Lord, and how great is Your beauty.

I am cheerful in You. Thou art beautiful, oh my love. And that day shall the branch of the Lord be beautiful and glorious, and the fruit of the Earth shall be excellent and comely for them that are escaped of Israel.

I have likened the daughter of Zion to a comely and delicate woman.

I sleep pretty. I rest well. I get my beauty rest. Lord, heal me in the night hours when the night is quiet, and while my body is still, in the Name of Jesus.

I am fearfully and wonderfully made.

Lord, make me beautiful and well favored, like Rachel. Beautiful, like Bathsheba. Beautiful, like Esther. Beautiful to You, Father. Beautiful in the eyes of my beloved.

Lord, make me a person of good understanding and of a beautiful countenance.

Men

As for the beauty of man—

So, he sent for him and had him brought in. He was glowing with health and had a fine appearance and handsome features. Then the Lord said, "Rise and anoint him; this is the one." (1 Samuel 16:12 NIV)

For this is the mighty men of valor before the Lord, beautiful, handsome, manly men.

At that time Moses was born and was exceedingly handsome. He was nourished three months in his father's house. (Acts 7:20).

They were to be young men without physical defect, handsome in appearance, skilled in all wisdom, quick to learn, (Daniel 1:4a).

You are the most handsome of men; grace flows from your lips. Therefore God has blessed you forever, (Psalm 45:2).

Thank You, Lord even though you look on the inward, you make all things beautiful in their time.

Healing Sleep

God gives rest to His beloved, and I am beloved of God. Father, in the Name of Jesus, I reject nightmares, night terrors, sudden destruction, and worry.

Beauty rest is the amount of sleep needed to keep one looking young and beautiful, fresh and vibrant. Lord, give me the sleep that I need to feel and look healthy and attractive.

I sleep pretty and I rest well. I get my beauty rest. Lord, heal me in the night hours when all is quiet and while my body is still, in the Name of Jesus.

Lord, when my body and soul are at rest, my spirit is alive in You, then I can worship You, Lord, in Spirit and in Truth.

I pray the Lord to age gracefully, and the Lord gives me length of days. My life, my body, my soul is preserved from premature deterioration, from premature aging, from unseen incidents, accidents, stress, wear and tear.

Father, where I have already worn down or have been worn down, restore me again to divine health. Ratify Your divine health covenant with me, in the Name of Jesus.

Thank You, Father.

I command the *spirit of restoration* and peace upon my life now, in the Name of Jesus.

Warfare

Every agenda of darkness to inflict me with barrenness of any type, including infertility, scatter, in the Name of Jesus.

Oh Lord, guide me and satisfy my soul continually with goodness and good things, in the Name of Jesus.

Satanic agents and any evil implantation, anything that is not of my Father, anything that's in my body that is not of God, die, in the Name of Jesus.

Every arrow to disgrace, or *of* disgrace fired against me, backfire, in the Name of Jesus.

The favor of the Lord is life. Amen.

Any arrow of darkness fired to scatter my health, life, or beauty, backfire, in the Name of Jesus.

Lord, bind up my broken heart and heal every wound of my heart, in the Name of Jesus.

Lord, put an end to my suffering; bind every *spirit of pain*. Lord, I forbid that *spirit* from working in, on, or against my body ever again, in the Name of Jesus.

I refuse to be like a stream that goes dry. I bind every *desert spirit* and every spirit of barrenness, in the Name of Jesus. **Return to sender**.

Lord, give me thoughts of peace and not of evil, so that I think on good things of good report, virtue, love and goodness, in the Name of Jesus.

I shall start well and finish well in life, in education, in childbearing, in child rearing, in business, in love and family, in relationships, in marriage, in the Name of Jesus.

All my body parts work according to the divine plan and function of God.

All my lady parts work according to the plan and function of God.

(Men) All my manly parts work according to the divine plan and function of God.

(Women) My ovaries function well and are normal, in the Name of Jesus.

Estrogen levels in my body: you shall not slow down or stop, in the Name of Jesus.

My monthly cycle becomes regular and stays regular according to the time of life, in the Name of Jesus.

My monthly cycle, you shall not cease prematurely. You shall not be irregular, in the Name of Jesus.

Any entity seeking control over my cycle, I bind you, in the Name of Jesus.

Fear of menopause, die, in the Name of Jesus. Lord, give me grace to embrace every season of my life, in the Name of Jesus.

Uncomfortable symptoms of menopause expire, in the Name of Jesus.

I am not a victim of sleepless nights, by Fire, in the Name of Jesus.

I sleep pretty, I rest well. I get my beauty rest. Lord, heal me in the night hours when the night is quiet, and while my body is still, in the Name of Jesus.

I age gracefully and I claim every sweetness out of life, in the Name of Jesus.

My health shall not degenerate or deteriorate. I am NOT falling apart, in Jesus' Name.

Hot flashes die, in the Name of Jesus.

Electric touch from Heaven, resurrect my menses where it needs to be resurrected, in the Name of Jesus.

Any marital roadblock in my life scatter, in the Name of Jesus.

My womb, receive divine healing, in the Name of Jesus.

Dream attacks against my life stop by Fire. I bind you and command you to go to the Abyss from where there is no return, in the Name of Jesus.

Satanic seal in my body break, in the Name of Jesus.

God gives rest to His beloved; I am beloved of God.

He has put all my sins behind His back.

Father, forgive me of vanity and works of the flesh, but I do want to look my best always and represent the Kingdom in a positive way, in the Name of Jesus.

Lord, renew my strength, renew my strength to live, renew my strength and renew the joy of my life, in the Name of Jesus.

I bind every evil *spirit* trying to zap my strength or my energy, in the Name of Jesus.

Lord, renew the mitochondria in my body to create more energy from the foods that I eat. Repair any cell and mitochondrial damage that may have already occurred, in Jesus' Name.

Anything draining or siphoning my energy, stamina, or my get-up-and-go, I command you to stop struggling within me now, in the Name of Jesus. I command you to get up and go. Get up and get out of my body and out of my life, in the Name of Jesus.

I bind every strength-draining, energy-draining, life-draining, idea-draining, peace-draining, joy-draining, time-draining, and beauty-draining infirmity brought on by any evil, in the Name of Jesus. Lord rebuke them now, in Jesus' Name.

Every vampiric evil be bound now and cast out of my body and my life, in the Name of Jesus.

Every zombie *spirit* be bound now and cast out of my life, in the Name of Jesus.

I speak renewal and restoration to my physical body and to my soul, in the Name of Jesus.

Lord, You are the strength of my life. Anywhere in my body that is weak, Lord, strengthen, restore, repair, renew--, renew me, in the Name of Jesus.

Fat Demons

Father, if there's such a thing as a fat gene, does my family have it? When I look at my family and my old family photos, do I see this pattern?

Father, in the Name of Jesus, remove the curse of the fat gene from my family's molecular and DNA structure.

I cut, break, and I sever ties to the curse of the fat gene.

I break every evil covenant that allowed it to come into my family. I break the curse that exists because of the evil covenant. I bind the demons assigned to enforce the curse.

I break up every *fat demon* working against my body and my family's bloodline, in the Name of Jesus.

Lord, help me lose weight and manage my weight if I need to lose weight. Help me to gain weight if I need to gain weight.

Lord, thank You for a healthy weight, healthy BMI. My body, I command you to obey the Word of the Lord as it concerns size, taste, cravings, sleep and exercise, in the Name of Jesus.

Lord, let me always love the taste of water, in the Name of Jesus.

In the Name of Jesus, we exchange the garments of the slave, the garments of oppression, the garments and attitudes of *mammy*.

I reject the spiritual garments of heavy body fat, always jolly, laughing, people-pleasing--, we break the curse of *step-and-fetch*, in the Name of Jesus.

My soul, listen up: this body will not harbor inflammation. You will eat better. You will sleep. You will drink more water, will put down the junk food, junk beverages, and we will exercise and be healthy, in the Name of Jesus.

Gut Health

Father, thank You for divine health. Thank You for gut health. Thank you for proper metabolism, especially carbohydrate and fat metabolism.

Lord, thank You for healthy cortisol levels that do not randomly spike or dip, so I remain healthy, in the Name of Jesus.

Thank You, Lord that I'm fearfully and wonderfully made by the hand of God.

All organs, cells, and systems work efficiently and correctly in my body, in the Name of Jesus.

Digestive system, you will respond to food, water, and any beverage the way the Lord Jesus made you to respond, in the Name of Jesus.

Teeth, mouth, esophagus, stomach, liver, gallbladder, pancreas, intestines, kidneys, you all perform at top efficiency with absorption of nutrients and expulsion of unneeded waste material, in the Name of Jesus.

Every foreign nonfood, non-beverage, every poison or evil implantation in my body, burn by Holy Ghost Fire. I render you harmless to my system and readily expelled, in the Name of Jesus.

Healthy is beautiful, and since sleep is important and necessary for carbohydrate metabolism, I get my beauty rest at regular intervals, in the Name of Jesus.

I sleep pretty, I rest well, I get my beauty rest. Lord, heal me in the night hours when the night is quiet, while my body is still, in the Name of Jesus.

Any familial predisposition for unwanted weight gain Father, change it, in the Name of Jesus.

Lord, please restore my family line to your original concept of health and healthiness, in the Name of Jesus.

For my muscle health Father, give me strength, motivation and opportunity to exercise and move my body in a healthy way, in the Name of Jesus.

My mitochondrial health, increase and improve, in the Name of Jesus.

Lord, take away all the shame for being obese, in the Name of Jesus. I bind you, *spirit of shame.*

Lord, forgive me; Lord I ask Your forgiveness for my anger, in Jesus' Name.

Spirit of self-hatred leave, *spirit of doubt,* leave. *Spirit of shame,* leave. *Spirit of fear,* leave me. *Self- consciousness* leave; ignorance to my condition, leave. *Spirit of self-defeat,* leave, in Jesus Name.

Show us how to defeat all *Fat Demons*, Lord, in the Name of Jesus.

Lord, bind stress from our lives to counter **inflammatory fat**. I bind every stress and stressor in our lives. Stress: leave, in the Name of Jesus.

Lord, give us the habit of eating the best and best tasting foods for our genetic constitution, in the Name of Jesus.

Lord, I destroy every food addiction in Jesus' Name.

Lord, reset our bodies biologically, in the Name of Jesus.

Lord, stop the invisible things that cause us to eat and overeat. *Fat Demons*, I bind you all, I forbid you from working against me, in the Name of Jesus.

Lord, balance all my emotions, hormones, and anything else that drives hunger, appetite, excessive appetite, and/or greed, in the Name of Jesus.

Fat gene, I evict you and ban you from our family, and our children and our children's children to 1000 generations, in Jesus' Name.

In the Name of Jesus, I rebuke the curse of *mammy* off my family line. I stand in authority for my family, and I cut, break and burn the mammy curse off me and every female in my family line, in the Name of Jesus.

Fat cells--, you have been with me since I was a baby, be the right size now. Conform to the blueprint that the Lord intended for me when I was created and born, in the Name of Jesus.

I bind every stress and every entity that causes any stress in my life, in the Name of Jesus

Lord, help us all, in the Name of Jesus.

I pray for divine knowledge, Wisdom and understanding, for healthy eating, and also for dieting when necessary, in Jesus' Name.

I take authority over every form of genetic and self-induced eating disorders and issues to include bulimia, obesity, gout, anorexia, arteriosclerosis, and cancer, in the Name of Jesus.

I bind the *spirit of infirmity* and I cover my body, soul, and spirit with the Blood of Jesus.

Lord, give me self-control regarding fats, carbohydrates, sugar and salt to maintain a healthy, lovely body and good health, in the Name of Jesus.

I shall not defile my body with defiling things, defiling foods, or defiling activities, in the Name of Jesus. I take authority and dominion over substance abuse and drug addiction, in the Name of Jesus.

I reject and rebuke *spirit food* given to me in the dream, in the night, in the Spirit as it is defiling, and I will not eat that, in the Name of Jesus.

I shall not die, but I shall live and declare the goodness of the Lord in the land of the living.

Jesus, if any part of my digestive system is under attack, heal it. Make me whole, make me regular and efficient in metabolizing all types of foods including carbohydrates and sugars and any type of beverage, in the Name of Jesus.

Fat cells, you've been here since I was a baby; be the right size, conform to the blueprint that the Lord intended for me when I was created, in the Name of Jesus.

Lord, anything foreign in my body, anywhere in my body, in any cell or organ, be removed immediately by the power of the Blood of Jesus, in the Name of Jesus.

Spirit of infirmity--, any disease or disorder, you are not welcome in my life, neither in my body and cast out, in the Name of Jesus.

Any abnormal metabolism, including any entity responsible for abnormal or harmful weight loss or weight gain, I bind you and cast you out, in the Name of Jesus.

Any evil *spirit* entity affecting my GI tract, the Lord Jesus rebuke you, and I bind you, in the Name of Jesus.

I recover every organ from every evil altar, and all evil altars militating against my health, household, be they local, environmental, territorial, international, or remote, be roasted to ashes by Holy Ghost Fire.

Blow wind of God and whirlwind of God, blow away every infirmity, in the Name of Jesus.

I rest comfortably. Heartburn, gas, indigestion, acid reflux, diarrhea, constipation, IBS, any and every GI disorder, you have no place in my life.

Lord Jesus, send your healing Balm of Gilead to soothe and heal, in the Name of Jesus.

I sleep pretty. I rest well, I get my beauty rest. Lord, heal me in the night hours while my body is still, in the Name of Jesus.

Thank you for divine peace upon my life, business, and job, in the Name of Jesus.

Warfare 2

Every evil arrow, every witchcraft spell sent against my sleep, my rest, my health, my beauty, my success, family or life, I dip you in the Blood of Jesus and I declare: Back to Sender.

Every spell of confusion, hardship, difficulties, problems, poverty, waste, mediocrity, hindrance, torment, stagnation, backwardness, closed heaven, iron Earth, brassy Heaven, rejection, reproach, disfavor, useless hard work, financial death, dryness, diversion, no helper, no Mercy, yokes of displacement, substitution, losses, opposition, impossibility, destruction, death, sickness, decay, tribulation, and bitterness, abortion of good things in my life, frustration, disappointment, and failure, I bind you in the Name of Jesus, and I break every spell, enchantment, incantation, chant, affirmation, sorcery, and all evil magic against me, in the Name of Jesus.

Break! Break! Break!

Vagabond anointing, marriage failure, family discord, sexual perversion, gluttony, hunger, thirst, deafness, rain of dust, I break you off my life right now, in the Name of Jesus.

I break every evil covenant that allows you to alight, and I repent. Lord, forgive me for every sin of my own and for all my ancestors back to Adam and Eve, in the Name of Jesus.

I break every curse; I bind every demon that is in place to enforce every curse. I send you to the pit of hell where you came from.

Every evil thing that has happened to me, I undo it with the Blood of Jesus, in the Name of Jesus.

I seal every doorway, gate, portal, every dimensional access point that allowed any evil into my life, with the Blood of Jesus. Amen.

And I count it as done, and I rest at night, peacefully, beautifully, restfully.

I call upon you Jehovah Rapha, because You are my healer. Jesus Christ nailed my sicknesses and diseases and pain to the cross more than 2000 years ago, and I declare that my physical body must line up with God's eternal truth for my life.

Your Word says that by the stripes of Jesus, I was healed. The Bible says that He, Himself took our infirmities and bore our sicknesses. Thank You, Lord.

Any evil *spirit* or entity affecting my GI tract, the Lord, Jesus rebuke you. I bind you, in the Name of Jesus.

Any evil arrow I declare that you are extracted from any target on or near my body, my family, my household, my business, my marriage, my life. Return to sender, in the Name of Jesus.

Any evil altar sending out evil arrows be, crushed by the Thunder Hammer of God.

I dwell in safety and peace.

Shock and amazement of any nature, you are not welcome in my life. I receive the peace of God that passes all understanding. (X2)

Neither torment, sudden terror, nor sudden destruction will have any effect on me. You will be far away from me, in the Name of Jesus.

Stress, I bind you, in the Name of Jesus.

Stress eating, I bind you, in the Name of Jesus

Eating my feelings and emotional eating, I bind you, in the Name of Jesus.

Emotional drinking to cope with stress, drinking to excess, I bind you, in the Name of Jesus.

Comfort foods that don't comfort, lose your effect on me, in the Name of Jesus.

Lord, restore my emotions, my soul, so that I do not seek natural things in my life that need spiritual healing.

Heal me, Lord, and I shall be healed.

The Lord restores my soul, in the Name of Jesus. Amen.

Pool of Siloam

To my ears and eyes and taste buds--, all other sense organs-- Lord, Your Word is health into my flesh and strength to my bones.

Lord, thank You for inviting and hearing these prayers today, in the Name of Jesus.

Lord, give me bright eyes, eagle's eyes, spiritual eyes, keen eyes, keen eyesight in the natural and in the Spirit.

Lord, give me clear eyes, beautiful rest and no bloodshot eyes, in the Name of Jesus.

And Lord, where my sight is blurred or dim, heal me, in Jesus' Name.

You said in Your Word that You forgive our sins and heal us of all our diseases, in the Name of Jesus. Lord, heal my eyes, my spiritual eyes, so that I can see through the tricks and traps of the enemy.

Lord, give me discernment to spot a masquerade; give me eyes to recognize, eyes to recognize a false angel of light, and not to be deceived, in the Name of Jesus.

In my natural eyes, Lord, I command health and healing and wholeness over my eyes, in the Name of Jesus.

Eyes--, vision restored to 100% like Bartimaeus, fill our eyes, Lord, with light. And the Lord opens the eyes of the blind. The Lord raises up those who are bowed down.

I've never seen the righteous forsaken or their seed beg bread, in the Name of Jesus.

Lord, You will never leave me or forsake me, in the Name of Jesus.

The Spirit of the Lord is upon me because He has anointed me to preach the Gospel to the poor. He sent me to proclaim the release of the captives and recovery of sight to the blind, to set free those who are oppressed. To open their eyes that they may turn from darkness to light and from the dominion of Satan to God, that they may receive forgiveness of sins and an inheritance among those who have been sanctified by faith in Me, says the Lord.

The lamp of the body is the eye. Lord let my eyes be sound spiritually and naturally, in the Name of Jesus, that my whole body is filled with light, in Jesus' Name.

Lord, rebuke all darkness from my life, give me spiritual eyes to see. Until that time see for me and give me awareness to know when I need to go left, go right, and when I need to pray. Holy Spirit be my intercessor, Jesus Christ our Great Intercessor.

Lord, I bind the *spirit of fear* and any hindrance to receiving spiritual sight, in Jesus' Name.

And Lord my healer, heal my eyes, in the Name of Jesus in the natural.

Lord, heal every disease, every disorder, and all age-related eye diseases such as age-related macular degeneration, cataract, diabetic retinopathy and glaucoma, thyroid eye disease, uncorrected, refractive errors--, near sightedness, far sightedness, corneal opacity. Trachoma, CVI or cortical cerebral visual impairment, any intracranial hypertension, any hypertension, diabetes, retinitis pigmentosa or retinopathies, any vision loss to include eye trauma, any disease or disorder that affects the eyes, any blockage of blood flow to or from the retina, retinal artery occlusion or retinal vein occlusion, retinal detachment.

Any eye pain or discomfort, dry eye disease, sinus pain, infections, headaches, migraines. Heal me Lord; I shall be healed, in the Name of Jesus.

Lazy eye, astigmatism, color blindness, night blindness, dry eye, floaters, pink eye, any cornea disorders, any eye styes, and nystagmus. Optic nerve atrophy--, any eye deterioration. Heal me Lord, and I shall be healed, in Jesus' Name.

Lord, I ask You to all me to age gracefully in You, in the Name of Jesus.

Just a touch of the Master's Hand, a touch of the Great Physician and I'm healed and made whole, in the Name of Jesus. Thank You, Lord.

Central, general, and peripheral vision loss, I plead the Blood of Jesus--, by His stripes we were healed.

Lord, I bring the Pool of Siloam to all who need healing in their eyes, their vision, their sight. Restore perfect eyesight, in the Name of Jesus, wash and be made whole, wash and be made whole. Wash in the Pool of Siloam and be made whole, in the Name of Jesus.

Lord, fill our eyes with light. We are the light of the world. We are light made from light, in Jesus Christ. Amen.

Amazing Grace. Now we can see both naturally and in the Spirit.

Thank You, Lord for vision, sight and purpose, in the Name of Jesus.

Lord, make my eyes, eyes of peace, eyes of Your grace, eyes of truth, and I see good things all the days of my life.

Open my eyes so that I look up and see the Glory, the majesty, and the beauty of the Lord.

I look past the hills from whence cometh my help. My help comes from the Lord, because the Lord loves righteousness.

Hear This

Regarding my ears and my hearing, Lord, bless me with keen hearing, continual keen hearing, both in the natural and in the Spirit, in the Name of Jesus.

And Lord, where my hearing is diminished or even gone, restore me to form and function, in the Name of Jesus.

Tinnitus to be gone in the Name of Jesus. Buzzing, hissing, rushing, ringing of the ears, I bind you from any possible origin that you've come to me. I bind you and send you away from me forever, in the Name of Jesus.

I seal up all access points to you finding me ever again, lose my location and forget my name, in the Name of Jesus.

All damage done to the ears and the hearing, to all hearing apparatuses, to the brain, the nervous system, or any part of the body, I seek and speak the healing Grace of Jesus Christ, by Whose stripes, we are healed.

The damages are all reversed, and we are restored, Amen. Thank You, Lord.

Taste & Smell

Oh, taste and see that the Lord is good. He is sweet. My taste buds work optimally so that when I eat I am satisfied with the taste, the smell, the freshness, the complexity of food that's taken in, so I do not crave excessively or eat to excess, in the Name of Jesus.

Thank You, Lord, that all my senses work optimally in the Name of Jesus.

Spirit of infirmity, disease, disorder. You are not welcome in my life, nor in my body. I bind you, in the Name of Jesus.

I seal all these declarations across every timeline and dimension--, past, present and future, in the mighty Name of Jesus.

Thank You Father for answering these prayers, in the Name of Jesus.

Thank You Lord. Thank you Jesus. Thank you Holy Spirit. You are worthy. You are wise. You are mighty. You're victorious and wonderful. You're altogether lovely, the Bright and Morning Star. You are the Only Living God, the Lord our Banner, Jehovah Nissi. You are Truth, Peace, You are the love of my life. You are the Lord of my life. Mighty God.

Thank you for all things that pertain to life and to godliness.

Thank you for restoration and healing and wholeness, relationship, covenant, peace.

Amen & Amen.

Diabetes

I sleep pretty. I rest well. I get my beauty rest. Lord heal me in the night hours when the body is quiet and still, in the Name of Jesus.

Lord, thank You for the *health gene*, the gene of good health.

Lord, any predisposition of diabetes, cancer, alcoholism, or any other bad genes embedded in my bloodline, I bind and cast them out, in the Name of Jesus.

Lord, I bind any predisposition or proclivity to any bad disease, in the Name of Jesus. I cast it away from myself and my family, in the Name of Jesus.

Lord, I repent on behalf of the family member that introduced any curse to our bloodline, and I renounce it, I break it, and I ask for forgiveness.

Lord, I break it, and I ask Holy Ghost Fire to roast into ashes so that it has no effect on me or my family anymore, in the Name of Jesus.

I taste and see that the Lord is sweet. The sweetness of life is mine. It has not left, it will not leave me, in the Name of Jesus.

Diabetes, I bind you, in the Name of Jesus.

Lord, please come onto the battlefield of my life. You said that You would fight our battles and give us victory. Lord, make all my enemies surrender and give up in total defeat, in the Name of Jesus.

Lord, thank You for the power to stop all evil in my life. Lord, heal this land and give me a healthy, peaceful, perfect life, in You.

I am redeemed from the Curse of the Law. I'm free from all illnesses and diseases, by the stripes of Jesus, by the Blood of Jesus, in the Name of Jesus.

Beauty comes from within--, thank You, Lord.

Thank You Lord, for good health, so that my countenance is lovely and that You are pleased with me, in the Name of Jesus.

My body system: reject diabetes, in the Name of Jesus.

Every agent of darkness assigned to afflict me with diabetes, die, in the Name of Jesus. Owner of every evil load, carry your own load, in the Name of Jesus.

Dream attacks against my soul, against my body, against my spirit, against my life, die, in the Name of Jesus.

My body works normally as the Lord Jesus intended.

My body absorbs sugar normally and metabolizes it normally, in the Name of Jesus.

My body chemistry and endocrine system work as God designed, in the Name of Jesus.

Starchy food in my body receives right treatment in my body and are metabolized properly, in Jesus' Name.

Carbohydrate-rich foods, processed foods, synthetic foods, non-foods masquerading as food, I reject you completely and lose all interest in you from this moment forward, in the Name of Jesus.

Negative genetic predispositions, I break your hold over my body and my family now, in the Name of Jesus.

I renounce and repent whatever my forefathers did to change the genetic DNA expression in our family from what God intended when He breathed life into our bloodline, in the Name of Jesus.

Heart disease as a result of diabetes, die, in the Name of Jesus.

Kidney disease as a result of diabetes, die, in the Name of Jesus.

Liver damage as a result of diabetes, stop by Fire, in the Name of Jesus.

Blindness as a result of diabetes, be reversed; be healed, in the Name of Jesus.

Slow healing in the body, I rebuke you.

My body, receive accelerated healing, in the Name of Jesus.

Pancreas and insulin hormones in my body, work normally with efficiency as God intended, in the Name of Jesus.

Diabetes: you shall not kill me, therefore you die, and I will live and I will remain in the land of the living and declare the goodness and the works of the Lord here in the land of the living, in the Name of Jesus.

Every symptom of diabetes in my body. Die, in the Name of Jesus.

Foods that cause diabetes you shall not lure me or tempt me; I reject you, in the Name of Jesus.

Spirit of uncontrolled appetite, leave me alone and die, in the Name of Jesus.

Spirit of satisfaction, I *loose* you in my life, in the Name of Jesus.

God said that He would satisfy us with good things, in Jesus' Name.

My finances shall not be wasted as a result of diabetes.

Oh Lord, save me from the power of sudden death.

And I apply the Blood of Jesus over the doorpost and lentils of my house, my body, and my heart. Angel of death, you must pass me by. You must pass over, in the Name of Jesus. I shall not die but live to declare the works of God.

Excess sugar in my body, melt by Fire.

Blood sugar levels, be balanced now, in the Name of Jesus, life is still sweet.

All organ systems recover from all diabetic damage, in the Name of Jesus.

I recover every one of my organs from every evil altar, in the Name of Jesus.

Evil altars be roasted. Holy Ghost Fire burn. Whirlwind of God, blow away every infirmity, in the Name of Jesus.

I call on you Jehovah Rapha because you are my healer. Jesus Christ nailed my sicknesses and diseases and pain to the cross more than 2000 years ago, and I declare that my physical body must line up with Your eternal truth. Amen.

Your Word says that by the stripes of Jesus I was healed.

The Bible says that He, Himself took our infirmities, and bore our sicknesses.

Thank You, Lord.

Your Word is health unto my flesh and strength to my bones. Thank You, Lord. You're the God that forgives all my iniquities and heals all my diseases.

You said in Your Word that the prayer of faith will save the sick, and the Lord will raise him up, and if he has committed any sin, it will be forgiven.

Thank You, Lord.

I declare that Jesus is Lord over this body, which is His temple and the temple of the Holy Spirit. I speak to every cancer, virus, bacteria, and other compromising enemy of my body, and I declare that you are now coming under the destructive and redemptive power of God.

I speak to every illness or ailment, disorder, disease, syndrome, or symptom, and I declare that I am supernaturally recovered, in the mighty Name of Jesus Christ.

I sleep pretty. I rest well. I get my beauty rest.

Lord, heal me in the night hours while the night is quiet and while my body is still, in the Name of Jesus.

Asthma

Lord, free my body, soul, and spirit from any and all captivity of the devil and his entities, so that everything about my mind, soul, body, and spirit is healed and made whole, in the Name of Jesus.

I speak to you, Asthma, and any other respiratory disease: you shall have no place in my life from this day on, in the Name of Jesus.

Touch me, Lord. Inhabit my life and my being, and keep all evil away from me, in the Name of Jesus.

I bear in my body the marks of the Lord Jesus Christ--, Satan, do not touch me. Do not touch any part of me. Not my soul, not my spirit, not my body, in the Name of Jesus. Hands off.

Allergies, coughing, sneezing, rhinitis, sudden difficulty in breathing, and tightness in the chest, Asthma, bow at the mention of the Name of Jesus, in the Name of Jesus, thank You Lord.

Asthma, and any other and every other respiratory disease, I bind you and cast you out, in Jesus Name.

It is a finished work against every marine entity causing asthma or breathing difficulties in my life, in the Name of Jesus.

Any and every evil entity responsible for bringing this into my life, I renounce you. I break all covenants made with you, either knowingly or unknowingly.

I declare that you must leave my life--, specifically spirit spouse--, aside from other torment, you bring asthma. You must leave and take your diseases with you. You must leave my life now and take your foul diseases with you, in the Name of Jesus. The Blood of Jesus is against you,

I breathe the breath of God. God has breathed into me to make **me** a living soul. You have no right to *my* air, oxygen, or breath, in the Name of Jesus.

Father, thank You for the prayer of faith whereby we may be healed, in the Name of Jesus.

Pneumonia. I break every evil covenant of my ancestors, going back at least 10 generations, but really to Adam and Eve on both sides of my family. I renounce evil and ungodly relationships that I may have participated in, and I renounce and denounce every evil covenant that opened the door for respiratory attack, including pneumonia or any other attack in my life, in the Name of Jesus.

Evil altars, be burned beyond recognition, in the Name of Jesus,

Any evil priest presiding at any evil altar be roasted to ashes, in the Name of Jesus. I bind all devils assigned to bring this and any curse into my life,

Lord, thank You for healing me, in Jesus' Name.

Ungodly, mutated genetic predisposition I break your hold over my body and my family now, in the Name of Jesus,

I renounce and repent of whatever my forefathers did to change the genetic or DNA expression in our family from what God intended when He breathed life into our bloodline--, I renounce and I denounce it and I repent of it. Lord, in the Name of Jesus,

I renounce. I repent of my own sin. Lord, please forgive me and remove *spirit spouse* from my life forever, in the Name of Jesus.

Lord, heal every symptom of asthma in my body, in the Name of Jesus. Every agent of darkness introducing sickness into my body, die, in the Name of Jesus.

My body, I release you from sickness and disease, in the Name of Jesus.

My soul shall not harbor the *spirit of sudden death*, in the Name of Jesus,

Every altar of darkness assigned against me, catch fire, in the Name of Jesus.

My airways receive strength and do not yield to evil ways, in the Name of Jesus.

My airways receive strength, in the Name of Jesus.

Oh Lord, lay Your hand of divine healing upon my life, in the Name of Jesus.

Owner of every evil load, take your load. It is not mine, carry your own load, it is not mine, carry your own load, in the Name of Jesus.

Every evil trap assigned against me, scatter, in the Name of Jesus.

Fear of sudden death, leave me alone, in the Name of Jesus.

I shall not die. My enemy shall die, in the Name of Jesus.

Every arrow of sudden death fired against me backfire, in the Name of Jesus.

I receive divine healing. I am well and healthy, in the Name of Jesus.

Every work of darkness against me, scatter, in the Name of Jesus.

My Father, see to my situation and heal me by Fire, in the Name of Jesus.

Every arrow that has resulted in sickness, disease, disorder, any symptom, backfire, in the Name of Jesus.

Blood of Jesus bring death to the agent of asthma in my body, in the Name of Jesus.

I shall not pass from sleep to death, in the Name of Jesus.

Anything in my environment that triggers asthma, die, in the Name of Jesus.

I receive complete healing and good health, in the Name of Jesus.

Oh Lord, renew and increase my bank account for Your goodness, in the Name of Jesus.

My body --do not cooperate with the works of darkness, in the Name of Jesus.

Every coven of darkness assigned to arrest my soul, scatter, in the Name of Jesus.

Every coven of darkness assigned to arrest or impact my health, scatter, in the Name of Jesus.

Father, heal me by Fire, in the Name of Jesus.

My breath shall not seize or cease as a result of asthma, in the Name of Jesus.

My breath shall praise the works of Jesus, not the works of Satan, in the Name of Jesus.

Every type of pneumonia: In the Name of Jesus be it viral, bacterial, or COVID, I proclaim and I speak to the body: Be healed, immediately, rise up and walk, in the Name of Jesus.

Spirits from hell that caused this infirmity, I bind you and I cast you out, return no more, in Jesus' Name.

All breathing disorders, COPD, asthma, cystic fibrosis, emphysema, lung cancer, any and every lung disease, disorder, symptom, mesothelioma, pulmonary hypertension and tuberculosis, you are cursed and you are bound, and you are cast away from me this day, in the Name of Jesus.

Backache & Neckache

Backache, neckache--, every pain attack from the pit of hell backfire, in the Name of Jesus.

Owner of every evil load, take your load. These responsibilities are not mine; you carry it, in the Name of Jesus.

I reject sickness and I claim divine healing, in the Name of Jesus.

Any sickness costing me money unnecessarily I bind you. Die, be gone, in the Name of Jesus.

I touch the hem of Jesus' garment and receive healing in the same hour. Lord, I receive my healing, in the Name of Jesus.

Every evil handwriting against me be blotted away by the Blood of Jesus. Balm of Gilead, heal me today, in the Name of Jesus.

Heal me Lord. I shall be healed in Jesus' Name.

Every agony of backache, neckache, shoulder ache or any other kind of ache disappear, in the Name of Jesus.

Every satanic instrument assigned against my health break, in the Name of Jesus.

My back, you are not assigned for evil. Therefore, receive your freedom today, in the Name of Jesus.

Every pain in my neck, every albatross around my neck be removed, in the Name of Jesus.

Every Rumpelstiltskin spell where I don't even know what the spell is, and I have to guess it--, the Holy Ghost knows and He gives me utterance and power to break your curse, your spell, your sorcery, right now, in the Name of Jesus.

Every arrow of sickness fired against me, backfire, in the Name of Jesus.

Every occult power working against me, die, in the Name of Jesus.

All joints, tendons, ligaments, and discs receive proper hydration, now. Receive restoration and wholeness and healing, now, in the Name of Jesus.

How beautiful are the feet with shoes. Oh, Prince's daughters, thy joints are like thighs, are like jewels and the work of thy hands of a cunning workman. How beautiful upon the mountains are the feet of them that bring good things that published the peace that bring up. Things good Tidings of good that published salvation that saith under Zion thy God reigneth.

Thank You, Lord, that every foot pain, every foot ache, every bunion, planter fasciitis, every possible foot disorder, every foot sore is healed by the Blood of Jesus, in the Name of Jesus.

Lord Jesus, rebuke the pain. I bind the *spirit of pain* over the feet, in the Name of Jesus.

Every arrow of darkness against my life, backfire. Arthritis, leave. Pneumonia, leave. Asthma, leave. Foot pain, leave. Neck pain, leave. Backaches, leave, leave, in the Name of Jesus.

Lord, I repent for myself and down my family line, where I've been too stubborn to act, too stubborn to move, or frozen in place when You said, GO!

Where we've been stiff-necked, Lord forgive me and my ancestors, in the Name of Jesus, and all result in changes in the way our DNA is expressed. Lord, change it back, please to pre-sin days when we were fluid and movable and obedient to You, in the Name of Jesus.

My joints--, receive deliverance by fire. My joints receive deliverance by fire. My joints receive deliverance by fire, in the Name of Jesus.

I refuse to be rendered useless with sickness, in the Name of Jesus.

Every symptom of arthritis in my life expire, in the Name of Jesus.

My lifestyle, obey the laws of healthy living, in the Name of Jesus.

Divine healing from above locate me by Fire in the Name of Jesus.

Every source of dream attack against my life, against my health, dry up, in the Name of Jesus

By Fire, by force I vomit up all evil consumption that is working against my joints, my joint health, my health in general, and my comfort in my body, in the Name of Jesus.

I shall not expire before my time, Jesus' Name.

Every pain as a result of arthritis, die, in Jesus' Name.

I bind the *spirit of pain*, I bind the *spirit of infirmity*.

Every spiritual obituary, organized for my sake, scatter, in the Name of Jesus.

Any evil rope, padlock, zip ties, string, binding, ribbon, cord, or other binding, natural, spiritual, or energetic, assigned to tie my legs or feet, ankles in the natural, and/or in the spirit, BREAK!, in the Name of Jesus.

My body joints receive deliverance from satanic captivity, in the Name of Jesus, Lord Jesus, send

Your mighty angels to bring me out of every captivity, in the Name of Jesus,

Every arrow of sluggishness fired against me from the pit of hell, backfire, in Jesus' Name.

Every power of wickedness after my life somersault and die, in the Name of Jesus.

Any arrow of car, roadway, or highway, accident or incident, die, in the Name of Jesus.

Satanic Ambulance assigned for my sake, catch fire, roast to ashes, in the Name of Jesus.

My body receive the resurrection power of Jesus Christ in Jesus' Name (X2, or more).

Healing Covenant

Father, I enter a lasting Healing Covenant with You, All evil *spirits* behind sicknesses and diseases are now bound and prevented from acting against me, in Jesus' Name.

Healing Covenant, take away every disease by the stripes of Jesus Christ and the Blood of the Cross at Calvary.

Under the Healing covenant, diseases and sicknesses cannot attack.

Thank You, Lord. Thank You, Lord.

Father, I enter into this Healing Covenant with You, in the Name of Jesus.

No evil *spirit* is effective against me any longer, in the Name of Jesus,

All evil is bound. Lord rebuke all evil and cast it out into outer darkness, into the pit of hell for early torment, in the Name of Jesus.

By the stripes of Jesus Christ and the Blood He shed on the Cross of Calvary, all sicknesses and diseases are rendered ineffective against me, in the Name of Jesus.

Spirit of infirmity, any disease, or disorder, you are not welcome in my life, neither in my body. Be bound, be cast out now, in the Name of Jesus.

I sleep for beauty, for rest, for renewal, for healing, in the Name of Jesus.

Inflammation & Infection

Inflammation and infection, you will not take a foothold in my life. I am not your candidate. I bear my body, the marks of the Lord Jesus, be bound and destroyed by Fire, in the Name of Jesus.

Inflammation is the start of every disease; you will not have a home here, in the Name of Jesus.

Inflammatory fat, I resist you, in the Name of Jesus.

Lord, give me Wisdom and will power to resist inflammatory causing foods and beverages, and instead, give me a taste for anti-inflammatory, healing, pH-restoring foods and beverages, in the Name of Jesus.

My soul, listen up: this body will not harbor inflammation. You will eat better. You will sleep, you will drink more water, will put down the junk food, junk beverages, and we will exercise and be healthy, in the Name of Jesus.

Thank You, Lord.

High Blood Pressure

People of God be made whole: Blood pressure, whether too low or too high, be made normal, in the Name of Jesus.

Thank You Lord, thank You Lord. Thank You, Lord, for making us impervious to high blood pressure as we surrender our life to Christ, as we remain in His righteousness.

Thank You that we can pray against the works of the devil and that we repaired by the Spirit of God coming into our life, we experience the Resurrection power, healing and deliverance power of the Almighty God. Thank You, Lord.

As a remedy for every poison, Lord, I repent. I confess all my sins and I become a part of Your Healing Covenant so that even if I take up anything deadly or poisonous, it shall not hurt me, in the Name of Jesus.

I cleanse my blood with the blood of Jesus and every untoward result of poisons or high blood pressure disappear from me now, in the Name of Jesus.

I filter sickness out of my blood and send it to the pit of hell, in the Name of Jesus. Back to sender.

Every satanic blood bank waiting for my blood, catch fire and burn to ashes, in the Name of Jesus.

I shall not suffer stroke in the Name of Jesus.

Confusion and sorrow shall not be my portion in old age, in the Name of Jesus. I age gracefully, gloriously, to the glory of God.

I reject all senior moments, in the Name of Jesus.

Every arrow of hypertension fired at me, backfire, in the Name of Jesus.

Every sudden death arrow, backfire, in Jesus' Name.

Every arrow of bad health, you will not swallow me or my finances, in Jesus' Name.

God, come with Your mighty power and expel every symptom of bad health in my life, in Jesus' Name.

Every injury of my heart, physical, spiritual, or emotional, receive the healing balm of Jesus Christ, in the Name of Jesus. Thank You, Lord, for binding up the broken hearted.

Cancer

Every evil seed in my life, die, in the Name of Jesus.

Every troubler that wants to trouble my soul, die in the Name of Jesus.

I shall not sleep the sleep of death, in the Name of Jesus.

My blood, be corrected by the Blood of Jesus.

Every obituary announcement in the Spirit is canceled now, in the Name of Jesus.

All growths, tumor, or cancer, I destroy you completely and immediately, in the Name of Jesus, by Fire, by force.

Every part of my body, by the Blood of Jesus you are healed and free of all cancer cells, from the head, the skin, the brain, to the soles of the feet--, every organ, every system, every cell in between.

My blood and every bodily fluid I speak perfect health to you, in the Name of Jesus. You must comply with the Word of God.(X3)

Any and every evil arrow sent against my health explode midair and never reach me, in the Name of Jesus.

All arrows from unrepentant evil, return to sender.

Any evil arrow out for death, find your sender. I'm not your candidate. 1000 may fall and it will not come to me, says the Word of the Lord. Amen.

Jesus is mightier than any disease or disorder. Cancer, you are rendered ineffective and harmless against me, in the Name of Jesus.

Blood of Jesus speak healing for me. Blood of Jesus answer every evil arrow for me.

Blood of Jesus answer every ancestral covenant for me, in the Name of Jesus.

Covenant of Healing with the Most High God I speak health and divine healing. Divine health and healing and restoration are mine, in Jesus' Name.

Lord, excise all evil implantations in my body with divine surgical equipment, in the Name of Jesus. Uproot every tumor, cyst, polyp, mole, growth, cancer cell, and other evil implantations in my body and life, in the Name of Jesus.

Lord, *loose* your Divine Carpenters to seek and find every disease, disorder, any evil implantation in my body and remove it. Heal, me Lord, and I shall be healed, in the Name of Jesus Christ.

Thank You, Lord for divine protection. Lord, keep the enemies, plots and plans from reaching my life and my body, in the Name of Jesus, Amen.

Headache

Any stress that leads to headache, I overcome you by Fire, in the Name of Jesus.

Every symptom of headache in my life, die, in the Name of Jesus.

Tensions that invite headache pack your load and go, in the Name of Jesus.

Any stressor that brings on headache or migraine, be bound and cast far away from me now, in Jesus' Name.

Any power assigned to attack me with headache, be afflicted with it yourself, in the Name of Jesus.

My head, I clear you. Receive deliverance from headache now, in the Name of Jesus.

Every evil handshake that causes sickness, backfire, in the Name of Jesus.

Every evil arrow sent to cause affliction and sickness backfire, in the Name of Jesus.

I shall not be a victim of the hospital or in the hospital, in the Name of Jesus.

Every spiritual attack that leads to untimely death, scatter, in the Name of Jesus.

I shall not lose my sight as a result of headache, in the Name of Jesus.

Lord, protect me from sudden death, in the Name of Jesus.

Arrow of sickness backfire. There is a Balm in Gilead. Lord, heal me today and I shall be healed, in the Name of Jesus.

I sleep pretty, I rest well. I get my beauty rest. Lord, heal me in the night hours while my body is still, in the Name of Jesus.

Reverse Beauty Curses & Skin Issues

Son of Righteousness with healing in Your wings, make me more like You day by day, more beautiful, as You, Lord, are altogether lovely.

I break every foul, evil beauty curse ever uttered against me, either on purpose or by any blind witch, in the Name of Jesus. (X2)

Lord, thank You for skin renewal, for beautiful, bountiful, hydrated skin, in the Name of Jesus,

Father, thank You for good water to drink.

Thank You for good nutrition, in the Name of Jesus.

Thank You for collagen, for skin renewal, naturally or with supplements, in Jesus' Name.

Lord, make my skin lovely like Your bride in the Book of the Revelation, without spot blemish or wrinkle, in the Name of Jesus,

Father, I bind the *spirit of vanity*. Let me be beautiful and lovely like You for You, and my Kingdom spouse, in the Name of Jesus.

Cells be renewed, turned over, made healthy and whole, in the Name of Jesus.

Fat cells, you have been here with me since I was a baby--, you, be the right size--, conform to the blueprint that the Lord intended for me when I was created, in Jesus' Name.

Lord, thank You for healing. Lord, if I ihave a need for from any surgical or medical procedure, and I command a termination of all evil activities of the enemy against my body, especially as it heals now in the Name of Jesus.

My skin cells, receive renewal. Receive healing from sun damage. Sun, you will not smite me. You will not smite me with UV rays again, in the Name of Jesus.

Lord, renew and heal all sunspots, liver spots, esoteric spots, moles, skin tags, warts, blemishes, acne, freckles.

I embrace all wanted beauty marks, including freckles and moles, but all unwanted moles and freckles, Lord, remove those and heal me, in the Name of Jesus.

Lord, heal every skin disease, leprosy, and vitiligo, in the Name of Jesus.

All skin follicles be unblocked and cleared of all oil plugs, bacteria and dead cells. Lord heal me from all acne, in the Name of Jesus.

All conditions and diseases that attack the hair follicles, I bind you and any entity causing alopecia, in the Name of Jesus.

Every skin disease or disorder such as rosacea causing dryness, itchiness, scratching, redness, swelling, cracking, weeping, crusting, scaling, and any entity causing atopic dermatitis, I bind you and I cast you out, in Jesus' Name. You will not hide. I see you-- get out. Get out, in the Name of Jesus.

Every disease or disorder such as pemphigus, causing blisters to the skin, you *unclean spirit,* causing epidermolysis bullosa--, . Get out. I bind you and cast you out. in the Name of Jesus, the Blood of Jesus is against you.

Acne inversa and all other diseases and disorders that cause pimple-like bumps or boils, tunnels or tracks under the skin, I break the curse of your inflammation. I break the cause of your inflammation, in the Name of Jesus.

Psoriasis, and any other dry and thickening scaliness of the skin. I bind you at your root. Come out with all your roots, in the Name of Jesus.

Any and every other disorder and disease that causes thick nails, painful calluses on the bottoms of feet, or any other place on the body, I bind and cast you out, in the Name of Jesus.

Renaud's phenomenon, I come against you with the Blood of Jesus.

Lord, thank You for healthy circulation. Heart and blood vessels send blood to the hands, and regularly and correctly, in the Name of Jesus.

Scleroderma-- every entity causing Scleroderma, in the name of Jesus, Die! Leave the body and cause no harm to skin, blood vessels, and organs. Lord, heal every body part that has been affected or harmed by this disease, in the Name of Jesus.

Vitiligo, I command you to reverse. Lord give me even and normal skin pigmentation, in Jesus' Name.

Lord, I rebuke and bind up all things that cause scars, blemishes, wrinkles, bruises, scratches, large pores, indentations, lesions where they should not be, Lord, heal and give us resources if necessary and proper treatment to receive healing for skin renewal, in the Name of Jesus,

I repent and rededicate my life to You, Lord Jesus, and I block out all evil marks, be they natural, spiritual, or energetic, by the Blood of Jesus.

All evil *spirits* traveling with evil marks, or as a result of evil marks, I bind you and. I cast you away from me.

Evil marks causing disfavor, disappointments, marital delay, poverty and financial setbacks, failure at the edge of breakthrough, untimely death, sickness and work emotions, hard work with little to nothing to show for it, I bind you, in the Name of Jesus.

Destiny helpers, come back to me, in the Name of Jesus.

Evil marks of failure and rejection in my life, I reject **you**, in the Name of Jesus.

Blood of Jesus wipe them away. Thank you, Lord.

Lord, I anoint myself every night with anointing oil before sleep. Thank You, Lord.

Heal me and I shall be healed.

I rest well. I sleep pretty, in the Name of Jesus, and the Lord heals me in the night hours while the body is still.

Any demonic *number* identifying me for destruction, catch fire, in the Name of Jesus.

All marks of hatred, rejection and reproach, die, in the Name of Jesus.

It is written from henceforth, Let no man trouble me, and I bear in my body the marks of the Lord Jesus, in the Name of Jesus. Satan, I'm not your slave or servant in any way, I'm a bondservant to Christ.

Satanic odor--, that evil smell scaring my helpers and my spouse away, die, in the Name of Jesus.

Anything in me scaring away good things in my life, die, in the Name of Jesus.

Lord, change my life for the best, in the Name of Jesus.

I render the power behind any satanic marks in my body, impotent, in the Name of Jesus,

Lord, take away every evil mark and every evil odor that brings me shame, disfavor, reproach, or disgrace, in the Name of Jesus.

Any ancestral powers using demonic blade to cut my skin in the spirit realm--, fail! Receive frustration and die, in the Name of Jesus.

Every strange mark sent to introduce bad luck or disappointments into my life be cancelled by the Blood of Jesus.

Every room of darkness where my case is decided Holy Ghost fire scatter the entire council of them by Fire, in the Name of Jesus.

Every ancestral evil mark programmed in from my body from the marine kingdom. You cannot hold me ransom; be wiped out by the Blood of Jesus. The Blood of Jesus is against you.

Lord, let the anointing of the Holy Ghost break every yoke of failure at the edge of breakthroughs caused by ancestral evil marks, in the Name of Jesus.

Every witchcraft mark upon my organs be nullified by the Blood of Jesus.

Every local evil power using a strange mark to monitor me, go blind by Fire, in the Name of Jesus.

Every evil using my body as a dumping ground in the spirit realm, be consumed by Fire, Jesus' Name.

Evil marks of fornication, marital delay, be cancelled by the Blood of Jesus. Satanic attacks against my life backfire, in Jesus' Name.

Lord, I ask for cell renewal and healing from any surgery and for proper recovery, and I command termination of all evil activities against me, in the Name of Jesus.

Thank You, Lord.

I sleep pretty, I rest well. I get my beauty rest. Lord, heal me in the night hours while the night is quiet and my body is still, in the Name of Jesus.

Lord, free my body, soul, and spirit from any and all captivity of the devil and his entities, so that everything about my mind, soul, body, and spirit will be healed and made whole, in the Name of Jesus.

Touch me, Lord, inhabit my life and my being, and keep all evil away from me, in Jesus' Name.

I bear my body the marks of the Lord Jesus Christ. Satan, do not touch me. Do not touch any part of me. Not my soul, not my spirit, not my body, in the Name of Jesus. Hands off!

Sleep loss, sleep deprivation and all resulting symptoms, I speak to you. You will not attack me anymore, in the Name of Jesus. Thank You, Lord.

My body, receive divine energy, in the Name of Jesus.

Whatever I've lost as a result of fatigue, I receive it back 1000-fold, in the Name of Jesus.

Wisdom to capture the day, Lord, let it find me. Let that Wisdom find me by Fire, in the Name of Jesus.

Lord, whatever I eat, allowed to give me strength, in the Name of Jesus.

Every energy robber in my life, die, in the Name of Jesus.

Lord, nullify every poison or every other weapon against my body, and have me to expel it or remove it spiritually, in the Name of Jesus.

Every arrow of sorrow fired against me, backfire to sender, in the Name of Jesus.

Any power that wants to make life difficult for me, die, in the Name of Jesus.

Blood in my own body receive divine healing now, in the Name of Jesus. Thank You, Lord. Thank You, Lord.

Heaven, disgrace every Satanic load frustrating me, break it off of me, in the Name of Jesus.

Women's Disorders

Regarding women's disorders such as ectopic pregnancy, the devil's attack on all pregnancies, I bind them, in the Name of Jesus.

All attacks on pregnancies, marriages, businesses, all confusion, inability to conceive, failure to menstruate, irregular menses, prolonged pregnancies, prolonged menses, any evil exchange. I break your power over me, in the Name of Jesus.

Thank You, Lord, hormonal balance is restored in the women of God and the people who receive Your deliverance, in the Name of Jesus.

Devil, we are weary of your attacks on women, in the Name of Jesus. We are weary of your attacks on women, and causing reproductive disorders such as barrenness, infertility, PCOS, evil spirit, every evil spirit interfering with my monthly cycle, you've lost all rights to my life --, Get out! I evict you now, in the Name of Jesus.

I renounce any and every evil covenant that has allowed any open door. I break every curse as a result of this, in the Name of Jesus, and I bind every demon assigned to enforce the curse, in the Name of Jesus.

Spirit spouse--, get out, in the Name of Jesus. I am married to the Lord Jesus Christ and never to you, in the Name of Jesus.

Evil implantations, any evil implantation that's not of God be divinely aborted now, in the Name of Jesus.

I break your evil arrow that comes to kill, steal, or destroy, in the Name of Jesus.

I pray against every evil deposit in my body. Burn, burn, burn by fire, in the Name of Jesus.

Destiny stealers, you will not have my destiny, in the Name of Jesus.

Star hijackers, you will not have my star, in the Name of Jesus

Future stealers, you will not have my future, in the Name of Jesus.

Evil implantations from the devil and his agents in the lives of innocent people, the Lord Jesus rebuke you and I declare by Fire, burn off--, burn, roast to ashes, in the Name of Jesus.

Any evil error that comes to kill still and destroy--, back to sender, in the Name of Jesus. Any coven that is close the gate of childbearing against me catch fire and burn to ashes, in the Name of Jesus.

Every padlock of darkness fashioned against me break to pieces, in the Name of Jesus.

Every prophet of infertility against my marriage, die, in the Name of Jesus.

My marriage, hear the Word of the Lord you shall not scatter, in the Name of Jesus.

Arrows sent against my fertility backfire, in the Name of Jesus.

I receive a new womb, in the Name of Jesus. Amen.

Witchcraft judgment against me, scattered, in the name of Jesus.

Satanic seal against my womb. Break, in the Name of Jesus.

Power to fill the Earth and subdue it, fall upon me now, in the Name of Jesus. (X3)

My womb, receive deliverance from the hand of darkness, in the Name of Jesus.

Oh Lord, bless me with children and cover my nakedness, in the Name of Jesus.

Every curse of infertility in my life break, in the Name of Jesus.

Every dream attack against my marriage, scatter, in the Name of Jesus.

Every seed of infertility in my body, die in the Name of Jesus.

Every arrow of miscarriage, fight against me, backfire in the Name of Jesus.

Spirit spouse, die in the Name of Jesus. Spirit children, die in the Name of Jesus, in any order--, just die.

Spirit spouse putting a covering over my face to make my natural, physical, real Kingdom husband not able to see me, die, in the Name of Jesus.

Lord, reveal me to my Kingdom spouse and reveal him to me, in the Name of Jesus.

Spirit spouse sent to make me look older than my real age, die, in the Name of Jesus.

Spirit children that make me appear to have children in the natural when I do not have children, and thereby repel suitors—die, in the Name of Jesus.

I break every evil covenant I break. I divorce every *spirit spouse*. I burn every spirit marriage certificate. Spirit spouse, I command you to get far away from me, spirit spouse, lose my location, forget my name, forget my coordinates, in the Name of Jesus.

The Blood of Jesus is against you. I am married to Jesus Christ. Amen.

Men's Disorders

Father, as it regards men's disorders, I pray for every disorder against the men of God and the men who *will be* men of God, by faith. I call them forth into the Kingdom, in the Name of Jesus.

Depression, anxiety, PTSD, trauma, bipolar disorder, adjustment disorder, borderline personality disorder, mood disorder, substance abuse, alcohol abuse, opioid abuse, prescription drug abuse, I break your power over the mind of God's people, in the Name of Jesus, by the Blood of Jesus.

Erectile dysfunction, I break your power over the men of God, in the Name of Jesus and I break any cause and I bind any cause that may have led to it such as vascular disease, thyroid imbalances, diabetes, alcoholism, hypertension, anxiety, stress, and depression, in the Name of Jesus.

Premature ejaculation, I bind your power over the men of God, in the Name of Jesus, and I break all underlying anxiety, in the Name of Jesus.

Delayed ejaculation, I break the power over the men of God with this disorder, in the Name of Jesus. I break the curse, and I bind the demon assigned to enforce it, and I ask for healing, Lord, for nerve damage and thyroid disease, in the Name of Jesus.

Lord, I ask for healing for Peyronie's disease in the Name of Jesus Lord.

Lord, give a proper balance to those with low T, low testosterone with a low libido, or ED--, Lord, and let them be restored to healthy and youthful levels, in the Name of Jesus,

Father, in the Name of Jesus Lord grant restoration and healing of low desire and disinterest, in the men of God and anything that may have caused it such as fear, anxiety, stress. I bind all these stressors, in the Name of Jesus.

Father, heal, all psychological issues. And all relationship troubles, in the Name of Jesus. Lord I ask for healing for all medical conditions as in diabetes, kidney disease, depression, and Parkinson's disease.

Lord, I ask that all medications be regulated by Your Holy Spirit and heal people so they don't need these medications, but if they do they will take everything decently and in order from prescription drugs, all nonprescription drugs, such as over the counter use Lord.

I bind all sorceries, and all demons sponsoring recreational and illegal use of drugs, in the Name of Jesus.

Lord, I bind chronic alcohol use in, the Name of Jesus. Thank You, Lord.

Lord, I pray for the men of God, that they will enjoy the wife of their youth, and let her satisfy them at all times, and they will drink waters from their own cisterns, in the Name of Jesus.

Lord, forgive all spilled seed, in the Name of Jesus.

Lord, balance testosterone, and all other hormonal levels, in the Name of Jesus.

Spirit of depression, heaviness, pining away, and *grief,* the Lord Jesus rebuke you. I bind all these oppressive *spirits,* in the Name of Jesus.

Lord, I pray for emotional healing and all people for inner healing, especially the men and women of God--, bind the spirits of *bitterness, unforgiveness* and all works of the flesh, I bind and cast them out.

Lord heal all impotence, ED, Low T and all other diseases of the reproductive system for the men of God.

Lord, I pray that everyone will have inner healing but also be clothed in their right mind, mentally. I come against the *spirit of insanity,* I bind you and I cast you out, in the Name of Jesus. Thank You, Lord.

Father, forgive me of all sins that have opened the door to any *spirit of insanity* or *madness*, in the Name of Jesus. Lord, I ask for Your Mercy. I ask for Your Mercy, here Lord, in the Name of Jesus.

And Lord, please heal us of all evil inheritance for consultation with *familiar spirits,* hypnotism, fortune telling, fortune reading, astrology, magic, witchcraft, and any other activity that may have led to insanity or madness.

Lord, take control of our lives in the Name of Jesus. I proclaim the mind of Christ, and let this mind be in me that was in Christ Jesus. Let this mind be in you that was in Christ Jesus, in Jesus' Name.

Lord, in the Name of Jesus. I pray for all that may have been born into evil ancestry, they may have been born into a family where insanity was part of their evil foundation. I break the curses off them, in the Name of Jesus and I proclaim the mind of Christ and that everyone is clothed in their right thinking and in their right mind, in the Name of Jesus, from this point on.

Nothing is too hard for you, Lord. Mental illness is not too hard for You to heal or heal and return the captivity of those who are suffering mental illness.

I declare that any exchange that's been done against their mind, against their brain, that it'll be reverted back again so they will have their right mind again, in the Name of Jesus.

Lord, You have given us the spirit of Love, Power and a sound mind, in the Name of Jesus.

Lord, relieve us, receive us, and retrieve us all from all evil captivity, in the Name of Jesus. Thank You, Lord.

Put us back to factory settings. Give us a proper self-image. Thank You, Lord, in the Name of Jesus.

Lord, thank You for healing us of all sexual perversions, in the Name of Jesus.

Kidney & Liver

Lord, I bind all kidney disease, in the Name of Jesus.

All evil inheritance, all evil covenants and curses be broken now, in the Name of Jesus.

All kidney disease and all other diseases that make a person look old while they're still young, Lord, reverse those effects, in the Name of Jesus.

Lord, make us whole again, heal us, renew us, in the Name of Jesus.

Thank You, Lord.

Lord, I bind up all *spirits of reproach* and *shame*, *disgrace* for anyone suffering this, in the Name of Jesus.

Lord, I bind up all disfavor, hatred and rejection and shame as a result of it all. Thank You, Lord. Thank You, Lord.

And as a result of kidney problems, Lord I bind up eating in the dream, sex in the dream any evil defilement in the dream.

I divorce every spirit spouse, especially from the marine Kingdom, in the Name of Jesus.

We rebuke and reject all weight gain from this disease and disorder, in the Name of Jesus.

Lord, where mankind may declare it is incurable, there's nothing too hard for You--, Lord Jesus, just a touch, just a touch from the Master, just a touch from the Great Physician and we will be healed.

Lord, regulate all menstrual problems related to kidney problems, in the Name of Jesus.

I sleep pretty and I get my rest. Lord, Heal me in the night hours while my body is still, in the Name of Jesus.

Healthy Sleep Positions

Lord, give me healthy sleep positions, give me healthy breathing... lord when I am well and I'm healthy, I can serve you and serve people of God all to your glory in the name of Jesus. We'll put us all back to proper factory settings where you how you intended us to be, in the Name of Jesus.

I sleep pretty Or give me pretty teeth, pretty smile, straight teeth, white teeth, healthy teeth. Gums. Healthy gums. No bleeding gums, no deep gum pockets. Permanent teeth that are easy to maintain and no evil or unsightly deposits, in the Name of Jesus.

Lord, remove, rebuke, the spirit of grinding and teeth clenching, bruxism, the gnashing of teeth, and Lord thank You for protection of my teeth so there are no chips, breakages, loss of enamel, dentin crowns, or fillings needed, in the Name of Jesus.

Lord, save me and rescue me from captivity so there's no cheek biting, no tongue biting, no fear, stress, fighinting or flailing and kicking in the night.

I sleep pretty. I rest well; there's no tangled or mangled hair, no hair loss, no hair theft. But, instead, Lord thank You for soft, luxurious, long, healthy, shiny, beautiful, thick, bouncy hair, in the Name of Jesus.

Father, some of the hairs on my head that You've numbered are gone. They're shortened or they're not growing. We're storing every hair follicle back to life. Every strand of hair, Strengthen every strand, in the Name of Jesus.

Lord, I speak to each hair's follicle and I say, Grow, perform glow. You were created for a purpose. Grow, perform glow, grow, in the Name of Jesus.

For the long hair is one's glory. And it's God's glory on the women and men, in the Name of Jesus: Grow Lord, I break all knots and rope, curses or any evil curse, any evil beauty curse as it pertains to hair, skin, teeth, and posture, in the Name of Jesus.

Redeem us all from lost sleep and sleep deprivation and the results of it, in the Name of Jesus, Amen.

Lord, we know you can heal. You can heal me individually. You can heal my entire family and take away all the diseases and all the curses off our bloodline, in the Name of Jesus.

And, Lord, thank You that I look nice, not vulgar, or inappropriate in my clothes, in the Name of Jesus.

Lord, make my veins healthy so there are no varicosities, in the Name of Jesus.

Lord, smooth my skin make me beautiful like You because You are altogether lovely and I'm created in Your image and likeness, in the Name of Jesus.

Lord, resume and renew skin tone, skin texture to smoothness, so there's no cellulite or crepey skin on my body, in the Name of Jesus.

Lord, thank You for healthy nails and cuticles. Healthy feet, that are fungus free,

Lord, give Your angels charge over me to keep me in all my ways so I don't even dash my foot upon a rock.

Lord, I bind up and cast out all beauty curses sent by evil human agents, jealous witches, blind witches, and every gray-collar curse. Lord, block and break every curse emanating from any evil ancestral altars and foundations, in the Name of Jesus.

Lord, break up, condemn and destroy all evil altars emanating against me, in the Name of Jesus.

For every evil priest has been assigned against me, Lord, will you assign the Lion of the Tribe of Judah against them, in the Name of Jesus.

Flow river of God, and wash away all that is not like You, not from You, not approved by You in Jesus' Name.

Thank You, Lord.

I call back my energy.

I call back all fragmented parts of myself.

I call *myself* out of captivity.

Lord, send Your ministering Spirits, Your mighty angels to assist me. Where I've been in captivity, that I may be free again, in the Name of Jesus.

Father, search all the land of the living and the dead for my lost parts. Put me back together again. Remember Me, Oh Lord.

Lord, free my body, soul, and spirit from any and all captivity, and all from the devil and his entities, so that everything about my mind, soul, body, and spirit will be healed and made whole, in the Name of Jesus.

Touch me, Lord, and inhabit my being, and keep all evil away from me, in the Name of Jesus.

I bear my body the marks of the Lord Jesus Christ, Satan. Do not touch me. Do not touch any part of me. Not my soul, not my spirit, not my body, in the Name of Jesus. Hands off!

I sleep pretty. I rest well. I get my beauty rest. Lord, heal me in the night hours while my body is still, in the Name of Jesus.

And I come against every beauty curse that has ever been uttered against me, or ever will be uttered against me. Blood of Jesus, answer for me and answer every evil summons, in the Name of Jesus.

Facial Diseases

I come against, every disease disorder and every entity that is promoting these diseases that can eat up God's beauty and glory.

God's beauty and glory should be reflecting through my life and through your life, and I speak beauty and loveliness to the face, in the Name of Jesus.

Lord, remove every evil mark on me that the enemy has placed, in the Name of Jesus.

Lord, thank You that I'm about to reap a bountiful harvest in You.

I bind and cast out any evil that is opposing You, and my successes, in the Name of Jesus.

I am in the Health Covenant with God, in the Name of Jesus.

Lord, get rid of everything evil that's inside of me, in the Name of Jesus.

Workings of my body I command the Fire of the Holy Ghost to pass through you, and I decree a purging in my organs and every part of my body, and I command every sickness and disease to come out and disappear forever, in the Name of Jesus.

I command the root of affliction in my body to dry up now, in the Name of Jesus.

Any evil power that is supporting sickness and disease in my body be disgraced.

You, stubborn Egyptian diseases assigned to mock my health--, you are finished. Die by Fire, by force, in the Name of Jesus.

The anointing that breaks the yokes of sickness and disease appear and break every yoke of sickness and disease in my body, in the Name of Jesus,

You, serpent of sickness in my body, come out and die immediately, in the Name of Jesus.

My bread and water is blessed and sanctified by God. Any power polluting my bread and water, drink poison and die, in the Name of Jesus.

I decree death unto every sickness and disease in my body, soul and spirit. *Spirit of untimely death* to the good things in my life, die without further discussion, in the Name of Jesus.

Blood of Jesus flow into my foundation and kill every evil deposit by Your power.

You, enemies of my health, get away from me and come back no more, in the Name of Jesus.

My body, refuse to respond to sickness again, in the Name of Jesus.

Let the redemption and the Resurrection power of the Blood of Jesus redeemed my life from destruction.

Any sin in my life promoting ill health, drink the blood of Jesus and die.

Every sickness and disease in my body I confront you with the Word of God. Flee now. By the power in the Word of God, I bring divine help, long life into my body, soul, and spirit.

I decree frustration into the powers of all ill health in my life,

Any power that is attacking me with sorrows, wounds, and weakness. You are illegal; die and die forever, in the Name of Jesus.

I pronounce death against every sickness that has vowed to waste my life, in the Name of Jesus.

Standing before You, Lord Jesus. Thank You, Lord. I receive my healing. I receive my healing, now, whether the devil likes it or not. Jesus, You bore my sickness and took away my infirmities. Therefore, I receive my healing. I refuse to be sick, in the Name of Jesus.

Father, Lord, send Your Word to take sickness and disease out of my body, in the Name of Jesus.

Hepatitis and any liver disease, any disease of the liver or kidneys, I command my healing to manifest and waste every ill health attack against my destiny.

I invoke the power of God to quicken every part of my body and my life. You, my life, receive the quickening power of the Word of God. I decree a flushing of destruction against every evil poison in my body, and I command the depths of my blood system to be healed, in the Name of Jesus.

I decree death of the poisons of the fiery serpents in my life.

Every serpentine venom in my system come out by Fire, in the Name of Jesus.

I look up to Jesus, the author and finisher of my faith, and I receive my healing.

Whether the devil likes it or not, every judgment of sickness and curse of death over my life is reversed now and converted to long life and divine prosperity, and I glorify God. Amen.

Oh Lord, by Your Mercy change my sickness to divine healing and good health,

Oh Lord, arise and pronounce me healed by force, against any demonic disease. Thank You, Lord.

Lord Jesus, fill me with divine health and perfect my health, in the Name of Jesus. Give me perfect healing and perfect my health, in the mighty Name of our Lord Jesus Christ.

I receive my healing and health today.

Any power standing against my healing and my health receive a divine shock; die, in the Name of Jesus.

Blood of Jesus flow into my foundation and purify my body, soul and spirit by your power, in the Name of Jesus.

Thank You, Lord.

I receive a crown of long life and divine health, in the mighty Name of Jesus Christ.

Every iniquity in my life, harboring any sickness in my life, receive the judgment fire of God.

I decree against every disease, germ, parasite, bacteria, fungus, virus, any evil plantation in my life, Lord let the redeeming power of God, redeem my health and frustrate every weakness in my system, in the Name of Jesus Christ.

By the power of the everlasting decree of God, I receive the power of God to renew my health, in the Name of Jesus Christ.

Oh Lord, arise in Your Mercy and satisfy and heal me. Bring me good health by Your Word, by the Word of God. Renew my health, in the Name of Jesus Christ.

Let the Word of the Lord Jesus renew my youth like the eagle's, in the mighty Name of Jesus Christ.

Blood of Jesus, arise and put an end to every weakness in my body, in the Name of Jesus Christ.

Lord, give me the power to obey Your Word to the end. I use the Word of God for my healing. Let it saturate my ears, eyes, and overtake my heart, in the Name of Jesus and heal me Lord, and I shall be healed.

I receive the power in the Word of God, that increases life and adds health to the flesh, in the Name of Jesus.

By the decree of the Lord, I command every grief, sorrow, and all manner of sickness in my life to disappear from my life, in the Name of Jesus.

Every evil wound in my body, soul, and spirit, I command you to die, by the decree of the Lord. Every bruise and chastisement of my peace be healed by the power of God.

Let the healing power of the stripes of Jesus manifest in every area of my life--, now, in the Name of Jesus.

I appear before the Lord Jesus for deliverance, in the Name of Jesus.

Let the anointed power, in the Word of God, bring health into my body, soul, and Spirit, now, in the Name of Jesus Christ,

By the decree of the Word of God. You-- infirmity, sicknesses, and diseases in my life, you must die, in the Name of Jesus. Your presence in my life is illegal because Jesus has taken you away centuries ago, in the Name of Jesus.

Every evil force that is out to frustrate my health, in the Name of Jesus, by the decree of God's Word, I claim my healing and health today.

Lord, Arise by your power and keep me in sound health, in the Name of Jesus Christ.

Every seat of pestilence, fever, cancer, inflammation, itching, madness, heart failure, and all other sicknesses planted in any area of my body, die, in the Name of Jesus,

Holy Ghost Fire, let everything evil in my body burn to ashes--, all named and unnamed sicknesses that are in it, in the Name of Jesus.

I destroy every curse of sickness in my body, in the Name of Jesus.

I decree against every serpent of pestilence that is trying to feed on my flesh or cause any sickness against me to consume me, I decree you must be consumed by Fire and roasted by Fire, in the Name of Jesus.

Heavenly Father, let Your consuming Fire burn to ashes every feverish demon in my life. Lord Jesus, quench every Serpentine inflammation in any area of my body, any burning in my life from any Satanic kingdom, drink the Blood of Jesus.

Any serpentine vomit in my life that is causing extreme burning in my body, dry up and die immediately.

Let every stubborn problem in my life, die, in the Name of Jesus.

Every enemy of my healing and health receive confusion and leave me alone, in the Name of Jesus.

I decree death to every sickness that is trying to reduce me to a walking corpse, in the Name of Jesus.

Any evil bird or witchcraft feeding on my flesh catch fire and burn to ashes, in the Name of Jesus. Lord, restore me. Thank You, Lord,

Any tormenting seasonal or long-standing sicknesses of the body, soul, and spirit, leave me immediately, in the Name of Jesus.

Blood of Jesus speak deliverance into my life, in the Name of Jesus.

Emotions

Lord, I ask for more inner healing, for emotional hurts, bitterness, unforgiveness, unmet needs, unhealed, hurts, chronic disappointment, *spirit of grief, spirit of sadness*. Lord, give us the oil of joy for mourning and beauty for ashes, in the Name of Jesus.

Lord, for any facial diseases, so we age gracefully.

Lord, we ask you to heal distortions, all limitations, all pain in the name of Jesus, my body, my life, my face, resist any disease that induces old age before it's time, in the Name of Jesus.

And Lord by Your Mercy, change my sickness to divine healing by and to good health, a rise and pronouncement healed by force, by Fire, in the Name of Jesus.

Oh Lord arise, and I will be healed by force and by fire of every and any demonic disorder disease that's trying to eat my body instead you able to eat yourself and die.

Any evil pronouncement against my health, Lord Jesus, reverse it, in the Name of Jesus. Amen.

I receive my healing and health today, in the Name of Jesus.

I sleep pretty, I rest well. I get my beauty rest. Lord, heal me in the night hours while my body is still, and I am quiet, in the Name of Jesus.

Lord, arise in Your power and keep me in sound health, in the Name of Jesus. Thank You, Lord.

I soak my star in the blood of Jesus all night, in the Name of Jesus.

My life is not hidden. It's not hidden to God. It is not hidden to man. It is not hidden to my Kingdom spouse.

I sleep pretty. I rest well. I get my beauty rest. I'm lovely to my beloved. I'm lovely to my Kingdom spouse.

I am in good health. I do as the Lord instructs joyfully, gladly, in the Name of Jesus.

My life is not hidden. There's no covering cast over me; it has been burned off by Holy Ghost Fire, in the Name of Jesus.

I declare the scroll of my life is open to the things of God and only the things of God. Only the things of God that are on it will come into my life. The Lord Jesus bind and rebuke and take away from me everything that's on any false calendar, evil calendar, evil scroll, evil time clock, or evil timeline for my life, and I walk only in the timing of God for my life. Amen.

Thank You, Lord, for divine favor and life and relationships and family and business.

Thank You, Lord, and every covering cast is burned off, in the Name of Jesus.

Thank You, Lord.

Brain & Mind

I age gracefully, in the Name of Jesus.

I release my brain from Satanic captivity, in the Name of Jesus.

Every arrow fired against my brain, backfire, in the Name of Jesus. Brain damage, my brain is not your candidate; therefore, you expire, in the Name of Jesus.

My brain, receive healing, in the Name of Jesus, so I am not a candidate for senior moments. Any evil nail assigned against my brain, be pulled out, be pulled off, in the Name of Jesus.

My brain, receive deliverance from every work of darkness, in the Name of Jesus. Thank You, Lord.

Every arrow of madness fired against my life, backfire, in the Name of Jesus. Thank You, Lord.

By Fire by force, my brain is delivered, in the Name of Jesus.

Spirit of forgetfulness: Leave me alone and die, in the Name of Jesus.

My brain--, reject dream attacks and masquerades in the Name of Jesus. Lord, bless me with super memory, with super brain, in the Name of Jesus.

My brain, I release you from every altar of darkness, in the Name of Jesus.

I shall not be a waste to my generation, in the Name of Jesus.

I sleep pretty. I rest well, I get my beauty rest. Lord Jesus, heal me in the night hours while the night is quiet and my body is still, in the Name of Jesus.

Sound health be to myself and to my Kingdom spouse, in the Name of Jesus.

Lord, You are lovely, and You proclaim that we are made in Your image, and in Your likeness.

Thou art beautiful, oh my love as Tirza, Comely as Jerusalem, terrible as an army with banners. The branch of the Lord is beautiful and glorious, the fruit of the earth excellent and comely. A daughter of Zion to a comely and delicate woman. The Lord has made everything beautiful in his time. Also he has set the world in their heart so that no man can find out the work that God maketh from the beginning to the end.

Lord, repair the ruined cities. Lord, repair the hurt organs, the ruined bodies, the wounded hearts, the marked and deformed and distorted people of God and attacked and manipulated body parts because of sin, captivity, disobedience and rebellion--, Lord, forgive us all, in the Name of Jesus.

So that we awake, and put on your strength, O Zion.

Awake, awake, put on thy strength, O Zion. Put on thy beautiful garments oh Jerusalem--, garments of beauty, garments of health, the garments of strength, garments of love and relationship. Garments of life. Garments of victorious life in God.

Let the backbone of sleepless nights in my life, break, in the Name of Jesus.

I disgrace every problem that is behind my lack of Peace of Mind, in the Name of Jesus.

Father, give me sound sleep and rest, in the Name of Jesus.

Every evil presence in my life, disappear, in the Name of Jesus. Blood of Jesus flow into my foundation and cleanse all evil pollution, in the Name of Jesus,

Any *spirit of death* and hell that is tormenting my life, I bind it and cast it out, in the Name of Jesus.

Lord, let diseases and germs in every area of my body die by Fire, in the Name of Jesus.

I receive the anointing for sound sleep, and Peace of Mind, in the Name of Jesus.

I dislodge evil forces that have invaded my life, in the Name of Jesus.

Any organ of my body that the devil has captured is now released by the Blood of Jesus, in the Name of Jesus.

Lord, let any battle that is going on against my life end to my favor, let it end in my favor, in the Name of Jesus.

I remove any evil power that is obstructing my divine peace, in the Name of Jesus.

Let every evil visitor in my life die, in the Name of Jesus.

Any strange fire that is burning in my life--, quench, in the Name of Jesus.

Let every serpent of darkness in the garden of my life die, in the Name of Jesus.

Any evil power that has captured my eyes, come out and die, in the Name of Jesus.

Enemies of my health are disgraced, in the Name of Jesus.

Any evil power that has captured my worship come out and die, in the Name of Jesus. I worship the Lord Jesus Christ and Him alone.

Any power sent to attack my sleep, die, in the Name of Jesus.

I dislodge every *monitoring spirit* that is detracting from my sleep, in the Name of Jesus.

Every arrow of sleepless nights that was fired into my life, backfire, in the Name of Jesus.

Every enemy of my brain, die, in the Name of Jesus. Let my mental storehouse receive peace and rest from God, in the Name of Jesus.

Any evil yoke in my life that is supporting my enemies, break, in the Name of Jesus.

I terminate the visitation of spiritual robbers and satanic liquidators to my life, in the Name of Jesus.

Any evil covenant that is linking me up with demons in the night, break, in the Name of Jesus.

Any curse of sleeplessness in my life, expire, in the Name of Jesus.

I kill demonic angels that are on assignment against me, in the Name of Jesus.

Any invitation that my ancestors have answered or have given the devil, I withdraw it immediately, in the Name of Jesus.

I command every demon that has stolen my sleep to release it by force, in the Name of Jesus.

Blood of Jesus, speak deliverance into my life by Fire, in the Name of Jesus.

Blood of Jesus, destroy any sin in my life that is robbing me of sleep, in the Name of Jesus.

Let the redeeming power of God deliver my eyes from sleeplessness, in the Name of Jesus.

Fire of God, burn every enemy of my sleep, in the Name of Jesus.

Every enemy of sound sleep, receive double destruction, in the Name of Jesus.

Let the raging fire of God burn every serpent of the night that is distracting and detracting from my sleep, in the Name of Jesus.

Any evil priest that is ministering against my sleep, may your wishes against me backfire, in the Name of Jesus.

Let any witch or wizard that has vowed to destroy my peace drink bitter destruction, in the Name of Jesus.

Every unbearable heat on my head and other parts of my body, go back to your sender, in the Name of Jesus.

Oh Lord, arise and give me sound sleep, in the Name of Jesus.

I sleep pretty, I rest well. I get my beauty rest.

Lord, heal me in the night hours while the night is quiet, while things are still, my body is still, in the Name of Jesus.

Thank You, Lord, for the gift of long life.

Thank You, Lord, for the gift of health.

Thank You, Lord, for the gift of a long, healthy life.

Thank You, Father, for preserving, protecting and providing for me. I thank You, Lord, for those who care and help us as we age gracefully, and in our senior years.

Thank You, Lord, that we do age gracefully.

And, Lord, let me serve You in my old age, even like Caleb, with consistency and fervency; I shall not be weak, frail, or sickly.

I can do all things through Christ which strengthens me.

I pray for knowledge and Wisdom for healthy old age, and senior years, and diet, in Jesus' Name.

My bones will be strong--, not porous, and I speak strength to my joints and bones and marrow, in the Name of Jesus.

I prophesy that fire is in my bones. I bind every geriatric disease, in Jesus' Name.

I declare that no one will take advantage of me in my golden years, or abuse or harm me in my older age, in the Name of Jesus.

And the Lord will give His angels charge over me to take care of me at all times, in Jesus' Name.

In my golden years, I will eat the good fruit from my labor. My children, friends and acquaintances shall not abandon me in old age.

I shall reap every good seed sown in my life. I am blessed and I shall be blessed in my old age, because I've been a blessing in my relationships, and with my children, to my children, friends and acquaintances.

I pray for proper knowledge and Wisdom and the memory to maintain a healthy lifestyle, especially for my teeth, bones, joints, brain, kidneys and heart. I pray for divine function and consistency in my daily physical exercises.

Let me and my work be a blessing to my children and generations in my old age.

Lord, let me be a source of godly instruction and counsel to generations behind me. The Lord shall be glorified, and I shall leave a legacy of the Gospel and a godly example because the Lord us my Helper. He's the author and the finisher of my faith.

There's nothing too hard for God.

Thank You, Lord, for this great blessing, and for hearing these prayers and answering them, in the Name of Jesus. Amen.

I sleep pretty, I rest well, I get my beauty rest and the Lord heals me in the night hours while the night is quiet, and my body is still, and at peace, in the Name of Jesus. Amen.

Dear Reader:

Thank you for purchasing and reading this prayer book. May the Lord bless you richly, heal your body and keep you always, in the Name of Jesus.

Shalom,

Dr. Marlene Miles

Other books by this author

AK: The Adventures of the Agape Kid

AMONG SOME THIEVES

Churchzilla, *The Wanna-Be, Supposed-to-be Bride of Christ*

Demons Hate Questions

Don't Refuse Me, Lord (4 book series)

Evil Touch

The Fold (4 book series)

> The Fold (Book 1)
>
> Name Your Seed (Book 2)
>
> The Poor Attitudes of Money (Book 3)
>
> Do Not Orphan Your Seed

got HEALING? Verses for Life

got LOVE? Verses for Life

got money?

How to Dental Assist

Let Me Have A Dollar's Worth

Man Safari, *The*

Marriage Ed. *Rules of Engagement & Marriage*

Made Perfect in Love

Power Money: Nine Times the Tithe

The Power of Wealth *(forthcoming)*

Seasons of Grief

Seasons of War *(forthcoming)*

The Spirit of Poverty *(forthcoming)*

Triangular Power *(series)*

Powers Above

SUNBLOCK

Do Not Swear by the Moon

STARSTRUCK

Warfare Prayer Against Poverty

When the Devourer is Rebuked

The Wilderness Romance *(3-book series)*

The Social Wilderness

The Sexual Wilderness

The Spiritual Wilderness

Journals & Devotionals by this author:

The Cool of the Day – Journal for times with God

He Hears Us, Prayer Journal in 4 different colors

I Have A Star, Dream Journal kids, teen, adult

I Have A Star, Guided Prayer Journal, Boy or Girl

J'ai une Etoile, Journal des Reves

Let Her Dream, Dream Journal in multiple colors

Men Shall Dream, Dream Journal, (blue or black)

My Favorite Prayers (multiple covers)

My Sowing Journal (in three different colors)

Tengo una Estrella, Diario de Sueños

Wise Counsel (Journal in 2 styles)

Illustrated children's books by this author:

Be the Lion (3-book series)

Big Dog (8-book series)

Do Not Say That to Me

Every Apple

Fluff the Clouds

I Love You All Over the World

Imma Dance

The Jump Rope

Kiss the Sun

The Masked Man

Not During a Pandemic

Push the Wind

Slide

Tangled Taffy

What If?

Wiggle, Wiggle; Giggle, Giggle

Worry About Yourself

You Did Not Say Goodbye to Me

www.ingramcontent.com/pod-product-compliance
Lightning Source LLC
Chambersburg PA
CBHW050529280326
41933CB00011B/1514